I0478705

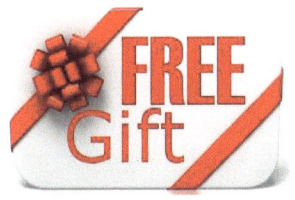

Want Priority Access to FREE eBooks Additional Materials for this Book?

As we release NEW eBooks, we offer them for FREE for a limited time. You will be the FIRST one to know when they are FREE. Join 1000's of insiders who are getting access to FREE Kindle book promotions weekly.

Click HERE for FREE additional material and FREE eBooks-
www.rictamilypublishing.com

Introduction

I want to thank you and congratulate you for downloading the book, *"**Anticancer Diet**: The Ultimate Guide in Fighting Cancer, Lowering Cancer Risks and Achieving Optimum Health"*.

This book contains proven steps and strategies on how you'll be able to fight cancer, lower cancer risks and achieve optimum health by following strategies and information relayed in this book.

This book will educate us on the following tips to fight cancer, to wit;

- The Truth behind Cancer;
- Preventing Cancer through Right Diet;
- How to Avoid Animal-Based Diet;
- How to Increase Fiber Intake;
- Saying No to Preservatives;
- Sorting Out Fats;
- Getting Raw Fruits and Vegetables Diet;
- Using Natural Soy;
- And How to Prepare Healthy Foods;

We hope that this book allows you to live a worry free life when it comes to enjoying your food.

Thanks again for downloading this book, I hope you enjoy it!

Chapter I: The Truth behind Cancer

The word "cancer" has become a threat to every individual and household. This disease has created fear and awareness. This word may sound simple, but it is really dangerous. Let us discover more about the disease.

Definition

According to the National Cancer Institute, cancer is a disease where abnormal cells divide uncontrollably and invade several tissues. These cells can affect other body parts through the lymph system and blood.

This is not just a single disease but is composed of many diseases and complications. Up to date, there are almost a hundred types of cancer, the majority of which are named after the organ of origin.

Origin

Our body consists of many cells, serving as our life's basic unit.

However, cancer starts in this very cell. Therefore, we should know how normal cells transform into cancerous cells.

There are many types of cells that can be found in our body. By nature, they grow and divide in a natural and controlled manner, in order to increase the cells in our bodies and maintain good health. Damaged or old cells die and are replaced with new cells.

The DNA of a certain cell can be changed or damaged, leading to a mutation that damages normal cell growth and its division. This alters the normal cell life. Cells do not die when the time comes for them and new cells are formed even if not needed. These new and unneeded cells will form a tumor, a mass of tissue that can be malignant (cancerous) or benign (noncancerous).

Levels of Cancer

The levels of cancer can be identified from its cause.

The two levels of cancer are the systemic level and the cellular level. The systemic level is the body's condition that allowed the cancer cell to deviate from its normal growth. On the other hand, the cellular level occurs once a healthy cell has turned cancerous.

Frequently Asked Questions

Q: Does a lump always signify cancer?

A: No. A lump may either be benign or malignant.

Q: Is it true that all of us have cancer cells?

A: No. According to Dr. Jennifer Loros, a professor of biochemistry and genetics at Dartmouth medical school, having to say this might be alarming. We all have cells that contain mutant proteins obtained from the damage of DNA.

Chapter II: Preventing Cancer through Diet

True to the famous cliché, "Prevention is better than cure", there are natural ways to prevent the risk of having a cancer. One of which is through healthy living and diet. Every person must consider eating a healthy diet regardless of family history related to cancer. Diet makes a major difference in the battle of this disease by increasing immunity.

Connection between Diet and Cancer

It is evident, there are many unavoidable health problems, however, you have major control over your own health, far more than you can imagine. Lifestyle choices affect the way cancer cells develop. A large percentage of deaths related to cancer root from lifestyle choices. Avoiding vices and addictions will surely help in staying healthy.

The foods that you eat and the ones you avoid having a powerful impact on your health. Unknown to you, you might be gradually fueling the cancer- cell production process through the food that you are eating. You should not ignore the nutrients and benefits that your diet might bring. Minimization of risks will be highly regarded by your discipline in diet.

Maintain a Healthy Weight

The best way to obtain your healthy weight is by conducting a test of Body Mass Index or BMI. This is the ratio between your weight and height. The need to reduce the risk of cancer gives a person a margin up to the score of 25. If you cannot comprehend the implication of your BMI, you can consult your doctor and seek an advice.

Moreover, maintaining a healthy weight reduces the tendency of complications such as diabetes and heart disease. If you are obese, you are prone to some types of cancer, such as colon, endometrium, breast, pancreas, esophagus and kidney. Also, excessive weight can aid in producing and circulating insulin and estrogen, which can stimulate the production of cancer-producing cells.

Chapter III: Avoiding an Animal-Based Diet

People want to eat protein rich foods such as meat. However, these kind of foods lacks essential nutrients that will help combat this disease. Also, the way of preparing and cooking animal- based foods are often dangerous to our health.

Relating Meat-Eating and Preparation to Cancer

Many studies have shown that eating meat in general increases the risk of cancer. These meats referred to include red meats such as pork, beef and processed meats. Yet, these enumerated meat products are not exclusive.

With regards to the preparation and cooking methods applied to the above mentioned foods, the temperature and duration required to achieve its best condition influence the compounds consisting the meat. Most often than not, stewing, poaching or boiling meat does not produce HCAs or Heterocyclic amines, chemicals that cause a mutation in the DNA. On the other hand, baking and oven- roasting produces a mediocre HCA. But the best ways of cooking such as broiling, barbecuing and roasting can produce a vast amount of HCAs which could really be dangerous to our health.

Aside from the preparation manner and time, duration is also an important factor. For example, a steak cooked in a well-done manner can form a higher carcinogenic compound compare to the "bloody" steak. However, one must also remember that undercooking meat is also inappropriate, which may cause infections and food poisoning.

Cancer Directly Related to Meat

Colorectal cancer, more commonly known as rectal cancer, colon cancer or bowel cancer, is caused by the unstoppable growth of cells in the colon or rectum or any part of the large intestines, causing it to spread abnormal cells to other parts of the body.

Having studied extensively, there is a conclusive evidence that processed meats and red meats contribute to the formation of this type of cancer. Though moderate, they can increase the risk of cancer acquisition.

Moreover, men who are fond of eating meat products have a higher risk of acquiring prostate cancer. The effects on women, however, are higher risk of suffering from breast cancer.

Chapter IV: Increasing Fiber Intake

Fiber is a form of carbohydrates our body finds hard to digest. Most of the carbohydrates can be broken down into molecules of sugar while fiber cannot. It passes through the body without undergoing the digestion process. It helps facilitate the use of sugars in the body and help ease hunger.

The Wonder of Fiber

Fiber works like magic in our bodies. More often than not, we cannot actually see or taste it. It is often found in roughages in plant's cell walls, which help combat diseases. Studies have shown that increased fiber consumption decreases the colorectal cancer risk. This is like a protective scheme, for fiber tends to add bulk to the digestive system, which shortens the duration of the waste traveling in the colon. Having to remove these wastes in the shortest time possible will eliminate the risk of carcinogens.

Protection that Fiber May Render

Protection from breast cancer can be achieved through fiber consumption. This is evidently true with the consumption of wheat bran and whole grains. The benefits of consuming fiber can be related to its low fat content. High consumption of dietary fats leads to a higher risk of catching the disease.

Moreover, studies have shown that fiber binds estrogen. High amounts of estrogen can be potentially harmful. The consumption of fiber aids in the removal of excessive estrogen from the body.

Fiber can also protect from throat, esophageal and mouth cancers. It can also provide protection against prostate cancer.

Fiber Sources and Weight Connection

Aside from providing protection and shortening the time of the waste removal process, fiber helps in regulating body weight. It acts like a sponge in the stomach, giving you a feeling of fullness, hence, hindering you to eat less.

Fiber can be found in (1) beans; (2) whole grains such as pasta, whole- wheat bread and the likes; (3) brown rice; (4) vegetables, primarily green leafy types, broccoli, spinach, and beans (5) berries, especially its skin and seeds; (6) bran cereal or any cereal with 5 grams of fiber per serving.

Chapter V: Say No to Preservatives

Preservatives are used to prolong the duration before the food spoils. They are added to foods, rendering them as an agent for hindering the decomposition process of microbes and stopping chemical change.

The Truth behind Preservatives

Before preservatives became popular, people died from eating sausage. This is attributable to Clostridium botulinum, the bacteria that causes the deadly botulism. In the early 20th century, researchers conducted a significant volume of research on the effect of nitrite, which is currently used as an ingredient in processed meats. Research revealed that nitrites can be linked to cancer formation.

Like any other matter, preservatives have the two sides of the coin. Through the development of preservatives, unhealthy foods such as processed foods and sugar treats have been enjoyed a long span of shelf life. However, on a brighter side, preservatives have also allowed enhanced access to healthy foods such as oils with unsaturated fats and whole-wheat products. Also, preservatives combat harmful microorganisms that act as food poisoning agents.

Preservatives and Cancer

In reference to a study published in 2012, a high dietary intake of nitrate in American women produced a high percentage of risk of acquiring ovarian cancer compared to those who enjoy a lower intake of nitrate.

Another research study proved that high consumption of nitrites derived from animal sources produces a higher probability of suffering from renal cell carcinoma. Nitrites can develop into nitrosamines, more popularly known as carcinogens.

In addition, the University of Hawaii (2005), conducted a study linking the risk of pancreatic cancer to processed meats.

Presence of Preservatives

Often, preservatives play a major part in the production of processed meats such as pepperoni, hot dogs, bacon, sausage, salami and red meat in frozen meals. These products are processed with carcinogenic content known as sodium nitrite. In addition, MSG or monosodium glutamate, can also be found in processed meats.

These harmful substances, along with other harmful chemicals, can be found in frozen pizza with meat, frozen meals containing meat, canned soups, pastas, ravioli, and kid's meals containing meat.

Chapter VI: Sorting Out Fats

The majority of the food we eat contains fat, good or bad. Some fats are good for your health while others are not. Completely eliminating fats in your diet is not possible. However, good fats can benefit the body, although they must be enjoyed in moderation.

Dietary fats contribute to the risk of cancer in two ways: the cells in a tumor need a low density lipoprotein to grow, hence, a diet that is low in LDL levels can keep cancer cells from growing. On the other hand, eating excessive fat stimulates the production of bile. Excessive bile stored in the large intestine for long durations can be transformed into a form of carcinogen, known as alcoholic acid.

Lower Consumption of Total Fat is Healthy

One must consume dietary fats, which are less than 20 percent of daily total food calories. For example, if you are aiming for a total caloric intake of 2,500, fat calories should be no more than 500.

Right Fats

The wrong kind of fats will trigger cancer more than eating excessive fats. Incidence of forming cancer is lower in cultures who have a high healthy fat diet, according to cancer researchers.

Some fats are not contributors to cancer, in fact, they contain anticancer properties. These "right fats" include unsaturated fats from plant- based foods, specifically legumes. Other good fats occur in omega -3 fatty acids found in seafood such as tuna and salmon, monounsaturated fats in vegetable oils such as olive oil, oils with Omega -3 rather than Omega- 6 such as that from pumpkin seeds, flax seeds, safflower, sunflower, canola, soybean and sesame seeds.

Research has shown that Eskimo women with a high concentration of Omega -3 in their diet have a lower tendency of acquiring breast cancer. The Omega- 3 fatty acids block the estrogen effect on breast cells, therefore, lowering the risk of transforming those cells into cancerous ones.

Avoid Bad Fats

Oils with high saturated fats shall be avoided, such as those in palm kernel, palm, cottonseed and coconut oil. Potential carcinogen compounds can also be found in hydrogenated fats, considered bad fats. Normal metabolism of the body can be interfered by fat molecules with a hydrogen component. This interference can set up a potentially cancerous change.

Hydrogenated fats are highly occurring in foods from fast-food restaurants, often acting as a preservative.

Chapter VII: Raw Fruits and Vegetables Diet

Since we were kids, our mothers would say fruits and vegetables are best for the health. Yes, if we had listened to what our mothers said, many diseases may have been avoided. Often, those common foods were taken for granted. Unfortunately, these foods are the primary needs of the body.

Reducing Cancer Risks

Hundreds of studies have been conducted regarding the link between cancer and diet, hence, they have arrived at the most common conclusion that eating a lot of vegetables and fruits lowers all cancer risks. Eating healthy foods tend to divert your appetite from fatty foods.

Phytochemicals are present in plant-based foods, which help the body combat cancer. There are five major compounds naturally found in plants that serve as a natural blocking agent of cancer. These are indoles, flavones, phenols, isothiocyanates and cummins. These agents prevent carcinogens from reaching the cells.

Identified vegetables that can lower cancer risk are broccoli, cabbage, mustard greens, kale, cauliflower and brussel sprouts. The above mentioned vegetables consist of cancer-protective biochemicals such as indoles, which reduce the risk of breast cancer; sulforaphane, which heightens immunity and hinders carcinogens from damaging healthy cells; and compounds that avoid the formation of nitrosamines.

Estimates from research show that eating leafy vegetables lowers the risk of acquiring colon and breast cancer by 40 percent. A vegetable salad-based main meal is among one of the healthiest eating habits. The phytoestrogens found in leafy vegetables can fill up the sites where potential malignant cells caused by estrogen can invade.

Anticancer Salad

We all want salads right? However, salads with a heavy cream dressing must be highly avoided. Salads should be plant- based and dressed with healthy oils in moderation. Vitamin C, Vitamin E and beta carotene, known to be antioxidants, constitute a synergistic effect when eaten together. So, mixing up fruits and vegetables with these compounds produces a higher anti-cancer effect, compared to individual intake.

Chapter VIII: Natural Soy

Soy produces heat-stable protein. This stability requires soy products to be cooked at high temperatures, and include items such as soy milk, tofu and textured vegetable protein.

Soy as Estrogen

Soy contains is flavones, which act as an estrogen. On the other hand, soy contains anti-estrogen properties. They can block natural estrogen by binding to the estrogen receptors. They can stop the estrogen formation in the fatty tissues and facilitate protein production that binds estrogen in the blood. They can also reduce the risk of cancer growth through their anti- inflammatory and anti- oxidant properties.

Soy acts as a protective agent against breast cancer and other hormone related cancers. A high concentration of soy in the diet will lessen the risk of acquiring breast cancer.

The Dark Side of Soy

Due to the popularity of soy as a "miracle food", the demand suddenly increased, and could not be catered to by the production of natural soy. The majority of the soy products in the markets today are not healthy. Most of them come from fermented soy and GMO soy that are contaminated with pesticides.

GMO and fermented soy are linked to digestive distress, malnutrition, thyroid dysfunction, cognitive decline, immune- system breakdown, reproductive disorders, heart disease and cancer. Also, it is linked to brain damage, infant abnormalities, kidney stones and fatal food allergies.

Soy as a Source of Protein

Natural soy contains plant protein, which is composed of magnesium, fiber, potassium, and other vitamins. They can be found in soy milk, miso, edamame and tofu.

Natural soy also contains essential amino acids that can aid in the body's vital functions. This might be the easiest way to achieve the required amino acids for people with food allergies or those adhering to a vegan diet. Hence, any excessive eating is not good, and all food should be, must be eaten in moderation.

The suggested daily soy consumption is three servings. A single serving may include one half cup of cooked soybeans, one third cup of tofu, and one half cup of edamame or one cup of soy milk.

Chapter IX: Preparing Healthy Foods

Food preparation is an important part of maintaining a healthy diet. Given the fact that you have chosen to follow the recommendations above, you must also have the knowledge regarding preparation of healthier meals.

Tips for Healthy Preparation

Here are some tips to follow for healthy preparation of meals. A household meal provider must keep cookbooks and recipes containing healthy cooking ideas. He or she must also be aware of choosing the parts of the meat to prepare. Loin, round meat and pork usually contain less fat, compared to other parts. With regards to poultry, leaner light meat from the breast is better than dark meat of the legs and thighs. You must also remove the skin. Which contains a lot of fat and cholesterol. You must also restrain from using excessive salt.

Making Seasonings Healthier

The meal provider must not use prepackaged mixes which contain excessive salt. Fresh herbs are encouraged. Pungent flavor can be obtained from the use of rosemary, marjoram and thyme. Citrus can be a substitute for commercial vinegars. However, vinegar works well with vegetables. Some vegetables and fruits give a burst of flavor when dried rather than fresh. These include chili peppers, currants, tomatoes, mushrooms, and cranberries.

Using Oil in Food Preparation

Liquid vegetable oils or nonfat cooking sprays are highly recommended. Whatever your purpose may be, choose oils lower in saturated fats, cholesterols and transfats like corn oil, olive oil, canola, sesame, safflower, sunflower, or soybean oil.

Other oils from plants are not recommended because of their high fat content such as palm oil, coconut oil, and palm kernel oil.

Healthy Cooking Methods

To avoid unnecessary fat and calories, frying must be avoided. Instead of frying, cooking methods should add minimum fat. These methods include stir-frying, which requires a small amount of oil; poaching, or boiling.

Sautéing is also advisable because it requires a small amount of oil. Steaming is also a healthy way to cook food.

Chapter X: Wellness Means Life

All of us want to live a long and healthy life. Yet, our choice of lifestyle influences our well-being. It is better to prevent diseases rather than curing them. Avoiding sickness is just a little sacrifice and taking necessary precautions. Why live a life with disease if you have the option not to?

Quotations Related to Wellness and Life

"Your attachment to unhealthy people and bad habits, which offer you no real control, is why you're spiritually dying and living a life out of balance."

Shannon L. Alder

"Health isn't about being "perfect" with food or exercise or herbs. Health is about balancing those things with your desires. It's about nourishing your spirit as well as your body."

Golda Poretsky

Physical fitness is not only one of the most important keys to a healthy body, it is the basis of dynamic and creative intellectual activity.

John F. Kennedy

Conclusion

Thank you again for downloading this book!

I hope this book was able to enlighten you more in assisting you to fight cancer, prevent it, and have a healthy life.

It is my hope that you'll also take advantage of the different substitutes available, to make sure that you're still getting your daily nutritional needs, but in a healthier, more cancer-free-friendly way.

Lastly, remember to enjoy everything in moderation and that even the good stuff, when taken too much, can also cause health issues.

Eat well and stay healthy!

Review Link

If you enjoyed this book, we would really appreciate it if you could leave us a positive REVIEW?

P.S. **You can <u>CLICK HERE</u> to go directly to the book page** and leave your review and/or purchase our other books above. Alternatively, you can copy and paste this address into your browser --- http://amzn.to/1wCj3OE

Preview of Liver Cleanse and Detox Diet

The Ultimate Guide on Cleansing the Body, Eliminating Toxins and Losing Weight!

You know what a liver is; there's no doubt about that. You know it can be found in the upper right portion of your abdomen, together with the gallbladder that shares some of its functions. It is the largest, and in many ways the most complex organ of the body. You may know how it works generally – for example, it helps cleanse the body of toxins.

But, do you exactly know how it functions, what vital roles it performs for our body to stay in excellent shape, and how important it is for it to be in top shape, too?

The liver performs many functions that aid in many essential body processes, that if it is allowed to malfunction, many of these very important processes will stop and put the whole body at a serious risk.

Digestion

The liver's main contribution in the digestion process involves its production of bile, a greenish-yellow and sticky fluid, which breaks down fats so that it can be easily absorbed or eliminated by the body. Bile allows for fats to be separated into small droplets so that they can be used as nutrients by the body.

Metabolism

The liver performs very important metabolic processes, especially in breaking down carbohydrates, lipids and proteins so that the body can make use of them. Carbohydrates are systematically broken down into glucose, which is stored in the form of glycogen. Hepatocytes are able to pack away and release glucose whenever the body needs it. Cholesterol and other forms of lipids are also produced by the hepatocytes to be utilized by cells throughout the body. Proteins are broken down into amino acids and undergo certain metabolic processes before they can be utilized as energy sources.

Storage

The liver absorbs glucose from the blood that passes through the hepatic portal vein and stores it as glycogen, which it can also readily release when needed by the body. The hepatocytes of the liver also absorb and store fats and other nutrients that allow the liver to keep the homeostasis of the body and to protect it from sudden spikes and drops of blood glucose levels.

Immunity

The liver also plays a vital function as an agent of the immune system of the body that helps eliminate and defend it from potentially toxic microorganisms through what is called the Kupffer cells. These cells help clean the blood passing through the hepatic portal system and the liver promptly, without having the need to launch automatic and harmful immune responses. This innate immune system also plays an important role in liver repair.

Detoxification

The liver acts as a filtering system that monitors and automatically remove potentially toxic and harmful substances before they get to the rest of the body. Through the enzymes in hepatocytes, many of these toxins such as drugs and alcohol are converted into inactive metabolites so that they do not cause any damage to the body. The liver also eliminates some hormones out of the body's circulation to keep homeostasis and hormone levels within limits.

The liver is not only the busiest organ in the body, but also the most overworked with so many of its functions involving metabolic and chemical processes. It is said to have a variety of over five hundred tasks vital to the overall health and optimal functioning of the body.

And with toxic elimination as one of its chief and primary functions, it is also the most stressed organs in the body which is a direct result of our modern lifestyle. It is unfortunate that we do not care enough as to the kinds of foreign substances that we allow our body to consume. Although, many of these substances such as environmental pollutants, pesticides, food additives, cosmetic ingredients, etc. are beyond our control, there are more than a few that we do have direct control, and that is through our diet, such as alcohol, drugs, caffeine and many more.

If we continue to ignore and fail to make the necessary lifestyle changes, we run the risk of damaging our liver and causing it to function inefficiently.

If you like this preview, then click here for the full story of this eBook!

Or go to: http://www.amazon.com/dp/B00QX9ENDC/

Check Out Our Other Books

[GOUT CURE: Your Ultimate and Comprehensive Guide in Treating Gout Permanently](#)

[ULTIMATE GUIDE TO FINANCIAL FREEDOM: Achieve Wealth, Attain Success and Manage Your Debt like the Rich!](#)

[GILGAMESH: King of Immortality – An Extra Biblical Proof for the Genesis Flood](#)

[HERBAL SOAP MAKING: How to Make Homemade Herbal Soaps that Clean and Nurture the Body!](#)

[PILATES FOR BEGINNERS: The Essential Guide to Total Body Fitness, Strong Muscles and Lean Body](#)

[TEETH HEALING THROUGH OIL PULLING: The Complete Guide to Natural Oral Care through the Benefits of Oil Pulling](#)

[THE AD: A Mail-Order Bride Romance Series](#)

[10 THINGS YOU NEED TO KNOW ABOUT EBOLA: Facts about the Virus, Symptoms, Quarantine and Prevention](#)

Dedication

To our three blessings that have made RicTamily complete and continue to grow together in His loving embrace.

Disclaimer

The information in this book is in no way intended as medical advice. This book is not meant to be used, nor should it be used, to diagnose or treat any medical condition. The author disclaims responsibility for any adverse health effects that come in combination with the use of methods and suggestions presented in the book. The publisher and author are not responsible for any health or allergy needs that may require medical supervision and are not liable for any damages or negative consequences from any treatment, action, application or preparation, to any person reading or following the information in this book.